An Easy Way
To Understand
Diabetic Neuropathy

Also By Brian B Jacques

His very popular Series of Mini-Health Books includes:

- An Easy Way To Understand Eczema and Psoriasis
- An Easy Way To Understand Stress and Depression
- An Easy Way To Understand Vitamins and Minerals
- An Easy Way To Understand Parasites, Worms, Candida, Constipation & Detoxing
- An Easy Way To Understand Crohn's Disease and IBD
- An Easy Way To Understand Body Building For Men And Women
- An Easy Way To Understand Alzheimer's Disease
- An Easy Way To Understand Herpes
- An Easy Way To Understand Parkinson's Disease
- An Easy Way To Understand Autism
- An Easy Way To Understand Fibromyalgia
- An Easy Way To Understand Your Body Systems
- An Easy Way To Understand Erectile Dysfunction
- An Easy Way To Understand Heart Disease, High Blood Pressure & Stroke
- An Easy Way To Understand Detoxing For Men & Women
- An Easy Way To Understand Diabetic Neuropathy
- An Easy Way To Understand Aromatherapy & Essential Oils
- Herbs For Healing
- How To Lose Weight After 40
- How To Lose Weight And Maintain Your Ideal Weight Permanently
- Amino Acids & Enzymes—What Are They & Why Do You Need Them
- The Little A–Z Dictionary of Herbal Remedies
- The Magic Of Vitamins & Minerals
- Effective Methods To Stop Smoking
- Eat Wholefoods And Take Supplements—The Ultimate Lifestyle Guide
- Stress Busters Adult Coloring Book

All these books are available as Kindle Editions and many of these titles are available as print editions from Amazon.com. Many are also available for the Barnes and Noble "Nook".

An Easy Way
To Understand
Diabetic Neuropathy

Brian B Jacques

Wisdom For Life Media

Publisher: Wisdom For Life Media (www.wisdomforlifemedia.com)

While they have made every effort to verify the information provided in this publication, neither the author nor the publisher assumes any responsibility for errors in, omissions from, or different interpretation of the subject matter.

The information herein may be subject to varying laws, regulations, and practices in different areas, states and countries. The purchaser or reader assumes all responsibility for use of the information.

All information included within this book is for educational purposes only. The author and publishers do not attempt to diagnose or treat any medical conditions, be it to do with health, diet or exercise.

If you consider that you have any kind of medical condition, then, you should consult a qualified medical practitioner or doctor or qualified naturopathic doctor before starting any herbal, vitamin and/or mineral program or supplement regime, exercise or health training program or diet suggested in this book.

This book is not intended for anyone under the age of 18 years, nor is it intended for breast feeding or pregnant women, underweight people or anyone with eating disorders or a health condition that requires special diets or medical treatment.

The author and publishers disclaim any liability for any loss however caused by anyone using the information contained in this book.

ISBN - 13: 978-1974365197

ISBN - 10: 1974365190

Published in The United States of America.

"Education is the kindling of a flame, not the filling of a vessel." —Socrates

Contents

Acknowledgment

To the many people I have come into contact with throughout my life, whose belief in me has made everything possible and worthwhile.

Introduction

Until recently, only a very few people had heard of diabetic neuropathy. Possibly the reason for this is because it only affected a small percentage of the population.

For those who had heard of it, the assumption was that it was only implicated in nerve damage to the legs and feet. However, this is only one type of neuropathy associated with diabetes.

Today, type 2 diabetes is a true epidemic; it is not contagious, but it is advancing so quickly that it appears like it is contagious.

Diabetic neuropathy is considered to be one of the more extreme symptoms of advanced diabetes. To the sufferer, it is one of the more apparent symptoms compared to other damage which is happening within the body.

Increased incidences of diabetic neuropathy are in line with increased rates of diagnosed diabetes.

Due to increased rates of diabetes being diagnosed worldwide, more resources are being directed to research into the disease. Public awareness is coming to the fore due to new education programs being developed. These programs are slowly creating a public awareness that type 2 diabetes is a disease associated with lifestyle choices.

It is not always comforting for a newly diagnosed type 2 diabetic to be informed that their condition is a result of previous diet and exercise choices.

There is however a positive outcome in that if they make changes in their diet and exercise program, then this can bring about changes in the disease; and as a result, many people have successfully "reversed" their diabetes disease.

This book will explain some of the causes and scope of diabetic neuropathy, in addition to explaining options for managing and overcoming symptoms.

There is also a strong emphasis on overcoming the underlying diabetic condition itself, which can have the effect of reducing current symptoms, and help prevent any further deterioration.

Chapter 1

What Is Diabetic Neuropathy

Type 2 Diabetes – an Overview

Diabetes is classified as a chronic disease which is becoming more and more common. One of the reasons for this is because people now tend to eat more processed and unnatural foods as opposed to eating more natural foods as once was the case. As a result of this, type 2 diabetes and other serious health conditions such as heart disease have become more common.

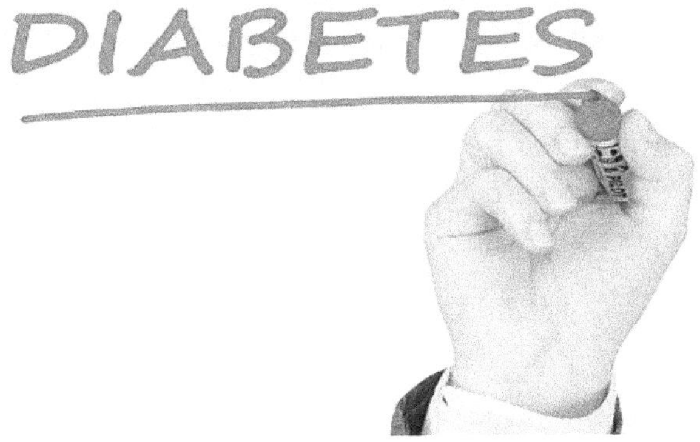

It seems that many people are unaware that high blood sugar levels in the body can lead to serious health condition.

The human body evolved with digesting proteins, fats and complex carbohydrates, which are digested and then release energy reasonably uniformly, at rates the body can use. Any excess not use by the body is stored as fat, which is then broken down for use when food is unavailable.

One of the big problems is the Western diet which is high in sugar, saturated fats, and often unnatural ingredients. All of this can lead to inflammation in the body, a condition called acidosis. Inflammation is a precursor for a variety of different diseases including heart disease, stroke, arthritis and diabetes; and as a diabetic condition worsens for the affected individual, diabetic neuropathy may become a serious issue for the sufferer. The Western diet is often linked to taste, convenience or both. The end result of this scenario—in addition to inflammation becoming an issue, is that the body's digestive system is constantly overloaded with an excessive sugar intake.

Each time there is an unnatural sugar overload—which can be as simple as consuming a can of soft drink—the body then releases the hormone insulin to process the sugar. What the body does not use immediately for energy it tries to store. Insulin is the primary hormone for removing excess sugar from the blood.

A pattern now starts to emerge. With the consumption of simple carbohydrates and sugar based foods and drinks on a regular basis, instead of an occasional basis, insulin is almost consistently present, instead of being occasionally present which is what our body's physiology was designed for. This is the beginning of the path to being diabetic as the body starts to become insensitive to insulin.

It is a vicious circle. To overcome this imbalance, the body releases increased amounts of insulin which has the effect of making the body more and more insulin resistant and an unfortunate consequence, the person now unfortunately becomes a type 2 diabetic.

Chapter 2

Is Reversal Possible

As of 2017, nerve damage resulting from continually high blood sugar levels in diabetics cannot at present be reversed. Current management of the condition includes: medication, lifestyle changes, exercise and diet.

As mentioned in the previous chapter, there are different types of diabetic neuropathy, and as a result, this condition can affect different parts the body. Current statistics show, that as many as 7 out of 10 people who develop diabetes will also suffer from nerve damage from the disease.

Reversing Peripheral Neuropathy in Mice

Although the condition is not reversible at present in humans, researchers at the University Of Virginia School Of Medicine, have succeeded in reversing peripheral diabetic neuropathy that was present in diabetic mice, which shows it may be possible to reverse the condition in the future. Remember, peripheral neuropathy is just one of four different types of this condition, the others being focal, proximal and also autonomic neuropathy.

As peripheral nerve damage is the most common type of neuropathy prevalent in diabetics, the results of the UVA researchers to succeed in reversing this very painful condition gives hope to diabetics who suffer from this condition.

Doctors Slobodan Todorovic and Vesna Jevtoviv-Todorovic discovered that high glucose levels which are present in diabetic neuropathy cases, results in some of the symptoms they do, as a result of the way they change how the body absorbs calcium.

In a healthy human body, correct levels of calcium move through pathways which allow absorption into nerve cells. Where a person suffers from peripheral neuropathy, these pathways are negatively affected. This results in too much calcium entering into the cells.

This excess calcium results in the affected cells becoming hyperactive, and this is what in many cases leads to the slight tingling sensations that are a common symptom of peripheral neuropathy. This over absorption of calcium is thought to be one of the factors that create excruciating pain which is on occasions experienced by diabetics who develop nerve damage associated with the disease.

Of particular note, the researchers were successful at reversing peripheral nerve damage in diabetic mice using a naturally occurring substance that is found in animals and humans.

The Problem with Current Diabetic Neuropathy Treatments

A word of caution though, human trials have not yet been started, and further research still needs to be undertaken to ascertain if this would be an effective way to go to treat and reverse this diabetic condition in the future.

Although at the present time symptoms which are associated with diabetic nerve damage can be treated and managed, there is potentially a problem. Quite a few of the medications which are successful in reducing or eliminating symptoms from diabetic nerve damage can create addiction problems in some patients.

In addition, some patients prefer to cope with the pain that is associated with diabetic neuropathy rather than feel tired, sleepy and experience poor energy throughout the day; which is often a side effect of several of the medications which are commonly prescribed.

To sum up, the fact that researchers have been able to reverse this condition in mice when it was previously thought that this was a condition for life, is very encouraging news. Mice are frequently used in all laboratory experiments because many of their internal processes bear similarities to humans.

There is hope that in the future this research will lead to a successful reversal of peripheral neuropathy in humans. In the meantime, diabetics have to rely on the treatments presently available which assist them in managing this and other forms of diabetic related nerve damage.

Chapter 3

Does It Ever Go Into Remission

It must be remembered, that the nerve damage associated with diabetic neuropathy is long-term. It occurs because of a constantly elevated blood sugar level. One of the most frequent symptoms of diabetic nerve damage is a lack of sensation or tingling in the feet.

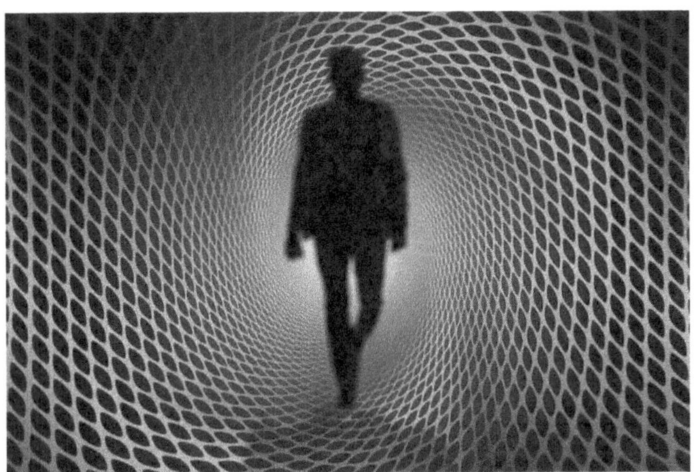

This lack of sensation in the feet can result in physical injuries that occur with something as simple as walking. If left untreated this condition often causes the development of ulcers and infections and in extreme cases can lead to amputation of the foot or lower leg.

Of particular concern, is the long-term effect of high blood sugar levels which causes nerve damage in diabetics. In many cases this does not usually present itself for several years—sometimes as many as 20 years can go by after a diabetic diagnosis has been determined. In some cases, pain can be so severe that it causes total immobility.

Interestingly, with many of the symptoms which are associated with diabetic neuropathy, there is no pain. Double vision can occur from focal diabetic neuropathy; or nausea may be experienced, possibly from an upset stomach or other digestive problems if autonomic neuropathy is identified. In both these cases there may be no pain at all.

Long-Term, Irreversible Diabetic Neuropathy is Possibly Treatable

Diabetic nerve damage and the many symptoms that are associated with it are irreversible at the present time. Whilst there has been research which shows the condition can be reversed in mice, as mentioned in a previous chapter, this research is only associated with peripheral neuropathy. Focal, proximal and autonomic forms of diabetic nerve damage have to date never been reversed in mice or other lab animals.

In all four types of neuropathy related to diabetes, effective treatments, but no reversal has to date been achieved in humans. The condition does not just go into remission; however, the symptoms can on occasions be managed whereby they are no longer a problem.

Controlling glucose levels can prevent further damage to the nervous system. This with a combination of diet, medication and exercise can control symptoms. The instance of neuropathy may be acute or chronic, meaning that symptoms disappear when the diabetes is under control, or persistent and reoccurring for long periods of time.

Treatment Protocols

It is important to realize that because diabetic neuropathy is irreversible does not mean that it cannot be treated. A diabetes condition can be reversible in some cases. And managing blood sugar levels is one of the best forms of treatment for both diabetes and the nerve damage associated with it, for up to 70% of diabetes sufferers.

Opioids may be prescribed if other treatments protocols are not successful. Unfortunately, many of the medications prescribed for treating diabetic neuropathy can cause serious side effects, including addiction that can affect quality of life.

Addiction must always be considered when pain relief medications are prescribed. Some medications can cause severe fatigue, a constant feeling of weakness and/or a lack of energy.

When the pain and other symptoms of diabetic neuropathy are minor in nature, patients can sometimes decide to put up with the symptoms, rather than experience the side effects associated with prescribed medications.

Having a healthy diet, linked with regular exercise and drinking lots of pure water (bottled water without gas is preferable to tap water, which contains various chemicals often misguidedly added by the local water company) throughout the day, and getting plenty of rest is a treatment protocol that can provide significant health benefits, and help in efficient management of neuropathy symptoms.

In some cases, a mild painkiller such as aspirin or paracetamol can provide significant symptoms relief. Antidepressant drugs may be prescribed to reduce physical pain. Nerve pain can be treated with such drugs as duloxetine, pregabalin and gabapentin.

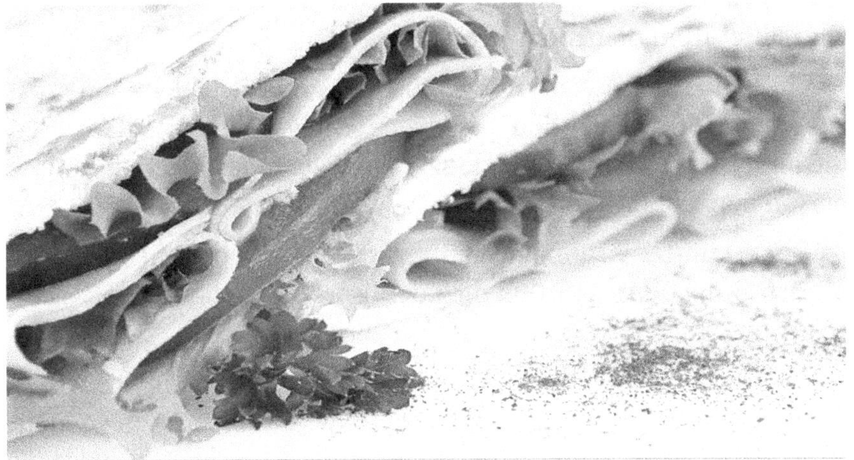

Chapter 4

Diet And What Foods Should Be Avoided

Everyone has certain foods that they avoid, often for reasons other than taste. It could be that there may be an uncomfortable experience if certain foods are consumed. As an example, tomatoes and tomato-based products may cause anxiety in some individuals and not in others.

There are individuals who can consume any quantity or type of food and not gain any weight. By comparison, other individuals may have to follow a very strict diet in order to not gain weight.

There are many ways that a diet may have a positive or negative effect on a person's health, and this is especially true with individuals who suffer from diabetic neuropathy.

When fat is mentioned and whether it is good or bad in food, then it is easy to form an opinion—everyone seems to have one. However, the important thing to remember is that, what may be good for one person may not be good for someone else.

Genetics and environment are intimately involved in the "makeup" of each individual, and this includes a person's reaction to certain foods and food types.

As an example, if a person is allergic to peanuts, then the person's body has developed a reaction to that type of food, so they would avoid eating it, knowing that if they did, it could cause serious discomfort.

For a person who is diagnosed with diabetic neuropathy, there are foods which should be avoided. In this instance, this is something where treatment should not be left solely in the hands of a Doctor.

Personal choices and actions regarding food intake, will potentially have the greatest positive impact on an individual's condition and symptoms.

If nerve damage has been caused as a result of a diabetic condition, then the following foods and liquids should be avoided if at all possible. Otherwise consuming them could aggravate the condition.

Monosodium Glutamate (MSG)

MSG is a highly dangerous flavor enhancer which is found in many different food products. In particular, it is often found in Chinese and Asian foods, as well as soups, frozen dinners, processed meats and canned vegetables.

What is often not realized is that it begins life as a salt—an ingredient that the majority of people consume far too much of. This salt is processed in such a way that it is converted to a flavor enhancer which is stimulating to the taste buds.

Monosodium glutamate has been implicated in various auto immune diseases, diabetes, as well as nerve damage in the brain, obesity and inflammation. Inflammation which is often caused by the "Western" diet is the precursor of most chronic diseases.

Monosodium glutamate is really bad news for diabetic neuropathy sufferers, as it has the ability to increase pain levels and further damage the nervous system. This is something that a person who already has a compromised nervous system does not want to happen.

Food manufacturers can be very cunning and hide the addition of MSG by using different names for it, such as: glutamic acid, hydrolyzed vegetable protein, sodium caseinate, textured soy protein, yeast extract and textured whey protein.

Alcohol

Alcohol, including wine and beer should be avoided if at all possible. The reason for this is because alcohol consumption is implicated in damage to the nervous system. Therefore, it is important to prevent any further damage to this vitally important body system.

Man-Made Sugar

Natural sugars which occur naturally in fruits and some vegetables are very good for you. In their structure, they contain various nutrients such as amino acids and enzymes, in addition to vitamins and minerals, all of which are required for healthy well-being.

By comparison, table sugar, as well as refined sugar and added sugars can be a pain trigger for individuals who suffer from diabetic neuropathy.

Like MSG mentioned above, food manufacturers can be cunning, and label man-made sugar in different ways. In fact they can use 100 different names instead of "sugar". Names such as: glucose, high-fructose corn syrup, fruit juice concentrates, corn sweetener, dextrose, fructose, in fact, any other ingredient which ends in "ose".

Aspartame

An artificial sweetener added to many processed foods, diet sodas, as well as some yogurts and candies, aspartame has the ability to heighten a person's pain sensitivity.

Researchers have discovered that when chronic pain sufferers eliminate diet soda from their diet, pain symptoms are reduced and often eliminated completely.

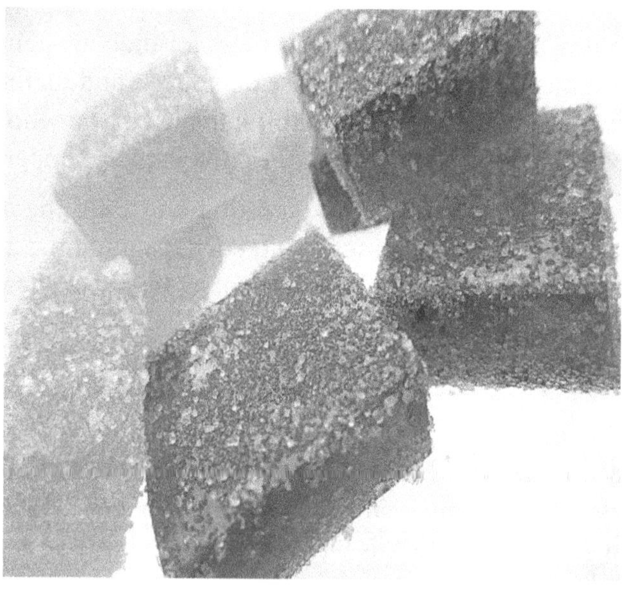

Chapter 5

Foods to Eat for a Good Diet

A person's diet is the greatest factor which contributes to whether glucose levels are normal, high or low. Therefore, some foods are better at managing a diabetic neuropathy condition than others.

As an example, eating bananas can help relieve stress and anxiety, whilst avoiding eating foods which spike blood sugar levels is a sensible way for managing a diabetic neuropathy condition.

Foods containing high glucose levels cause most of the damage in this type of neuropathy therefore, it is more beneficial to eat the majority of foods which are slowly absorbed into the bloodstream. These are foods which have a low glycemic index, or G.I.

Fresh fruits and vegetables fall into this category, which are eaten raw or have been lightly steamed, boiled or broiled. These types of foods are nutrient dense and are low in calories and carbohydrates. They take longer for the digestive system to process them, and as a result, they release glucose into the bloodstream in a controlled way;

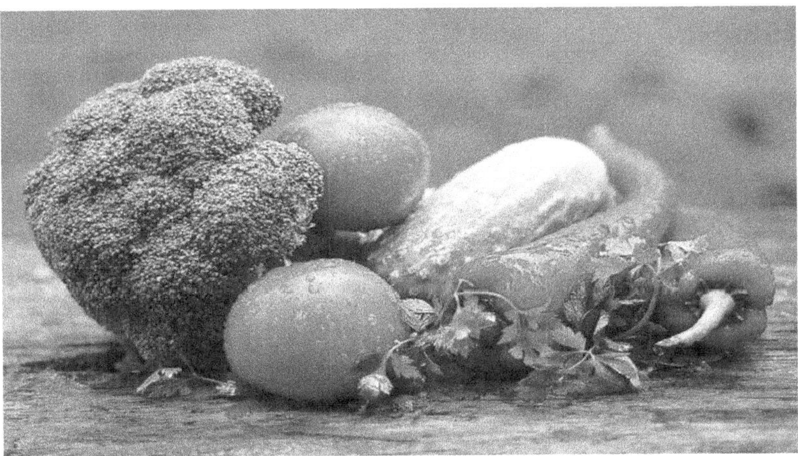

Since carbohydrates which are present in fruits and vegetables are known as complex carbohydrates. Therefore, their complexity and the benefits they provide to the body are determined by how they are constructed. As an example, broccoli and other cruciferous vegetables are classified as complex carbohydrates.

Sugar is called the King of simple carbohydrates. It is immediately released into the bloodstream, instead of in a steady and sustainable release.

Using the broccoli example mentioned above, with it being fibrous, it takes a long time to chew it therefore it creates a longer feeling of fullness after a meal, as opposed to when a meal consists mainly of simple carbohydrates. A good example is to sprinkle a small amount of sugar onto the tongue, which will take just a few seconds to be processed.

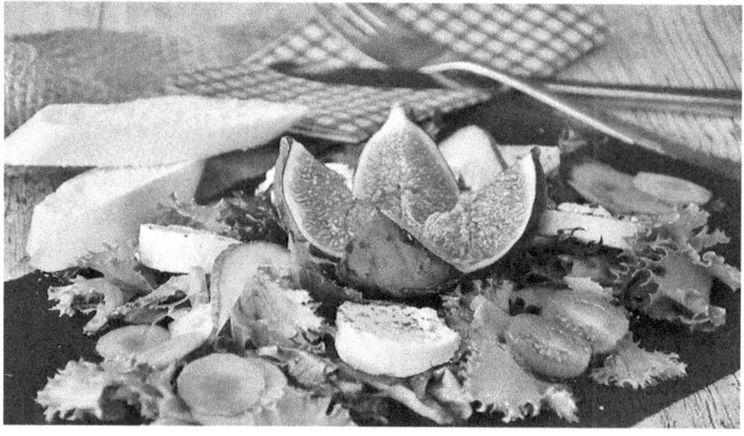

As complex carbohydrates take much longer for the body to digest them, there is no spike in blood sugar levels, which has the effect of providing better control of diabetic neuropathy symptoms.

High-fiber foods include split peas and lentils, black beans and figs. In addition, lima beans, artichokes, avocados and Asian pears are also high in fiber, as are chickpeas, nuts, okra, raspberries and blackberries, Brussels sprouts and oatmeal.

All the B vitamins are good for the nervous system. Good sources of B vitamins include eggs and liver, lentils, split peas and black beans mentioned earlier. Adding spinach, mushrooms, salmon and pine nuts will ensure that an individual gets the full range of different B vitamins.

It is important to remember that B vitamins are water soluble therefore they are easily excreted from the body, especially during times of body stress and anxiety. Taking a B vitamin supplement in a complex form is often advisable to ensure there is no dietary short-fall. I cover vitamins, minerals and essential fatty acids in greater detail in the following chapters.

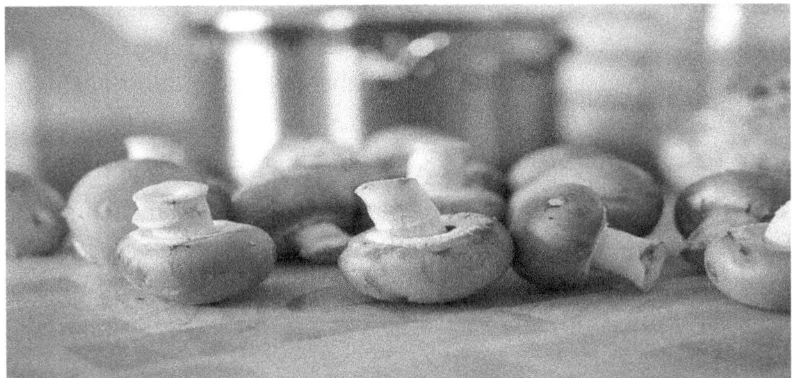

Keeping inflammation under control is crucial for managing diabetic neuropathy. Inflammation is the precursor for the majority of chronic diseases and illnesses. When the nervous system has been compromised by high levels of glucose, then, the nerves are more likely to be affected by inflammation.

Foods rich in omega-3 essential fatty acids such as oily fish including salmon, tuna, sardines or mackerel as well as flaxseed or flaxseed oil will have a cooling effect on any inflammatory condition.

Certain spices such as ginger, thyme and turmeric are useful for reducing pain signals and fighting inflammation. Cold pressed olive oil and resveratrol—a compound found largely in the skins of red grapes, which is thought to have antioxidant properties, are useful too.

Eating oily fish as mentioned above once or twice each week, as well as good servings of fruits and vegetables can have a positive effect on a diabetic neuropathy condition.

Drinking plenty of pure water—not tap water which is often loaded with unnecessary chemicals which has been added by a misguided water company—in addition to getting plenty of rest and regular exercise, if appropriate, will ensure that the body receives maximum benefits from the diet.

Chapter 6

Which Vitamins Are Good For You

Natural alternatives are available to help manage diabetic neuropathy, in much the same way as dietary changes are suggested to help prevent and reverse a diagnosis of diabetes. The quality of the diet can really assist in minimizing the effect of damage to the nervous system that has been caused by elevated glucose levels in the blood.

There are additionally certain vitamins, minerals and fatty acids which have proven effective for reducing the symptoms and pain associated with this type of nerve damage. The RDA or Recommended Daily Allowance of vitamins and minerals are prescribed for a healthy person.

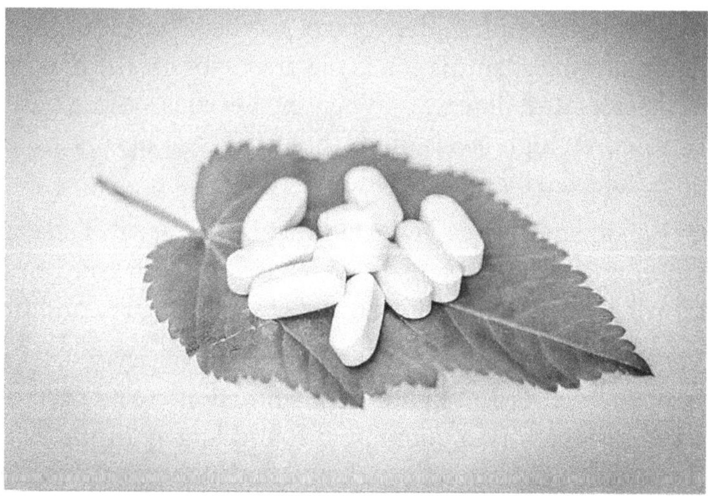

However, when a person is suffering from diabetes, their vitamin and mineral requirements will need to be increased to help deal with their condition. Unfortunately, many of the medications prescribed for diabetes and its various symptoms tend to either deplete vitamins and minerals from the body, or compromise the absorption of them.

For individuals suffering from diabetic neuropathy the effect is exacerbated. As an example, various antidepressant medications which may be prescribed for pain relief are amongst the worst for compromising vitamin and mineral uptake. It is always important for a person to ask their doctor if vitamin and mineral supplementation is appropriate in their particular case. Be advised that some vitamins, minerals and herbal treatments may interfere with any medications the individual may be taking.

Bear in mind that it may not always be possible to get all the necessary vitamins and minerals from the diet. The way the land is farmed, crops are grown, animals are reared, food is processed, stored and cooked, will all have a direct bearing on the end result. There is little wonder that experts today say that the body does not get all the necessary nutrients from the food that is eaten. A lot of the essential nutrients are lost along the way as evidenced by the growing and processing methods explained in this paragraph.

The answer is to take vitamin and mineral supplements along with essential fatty acids. And not just any vitamins and mineral supplements; any supplements that an individual takes should be natural, not synthetic. Natural vitamins and minerals have a life force within them; synthetic ones do not have this advantage, and as a result provide little nutritional value to the body.

By introducing a supplement program combined with a healthy diet consisting of various fruits, vegetables, nuts and berries, combined with an exercise program if possible and adequate rest and sleep, should ensure that the maximum health benefits are obtained.

It is also important to drink plenty of pure water (not tap water which in many cases is loaded with unnecessary chemicals) every day to assist in the transportation of all these essential nutrients to where they are needed in the body. Water is also important for assisting in the cleansing of toxins, impurities and waste from the body. This removal of waste material will help limit inflammation in the body, which has the benefit of reducing further nerve damage.

The following vitamins have the ability to slow down and stop the progression of neuropathy which has been caused by a high blood sugar intake.

There are two basic types of vitamin:

Fat soluble. These are stored in the body's fatty tissue and the liver. They reside in the body until they're needed—some for a few days and some for up to six months. Then special carriers take them to wherever they are needed. Vitamins A, D, E and K are all fat soluble.

Water soluble. These are different. When they are water-based they don't tend to get stored in the body as much but travel around in the blood stream. If they are not needed, then, they are expelled in the urine. That means they need to be replaced frequently. These vitamins include vitamin C and the big group of B vitamins—B1 (thiamine), B2 (riboflavin), B3 (niacin), B5 (pantothenic acid), B6 (pyridoxine), B7 (biotin), B9 (folic acid) and B12 (cyanocobalamin), B vitamins are especially important because they not only produce energy but also red blood cells which carry oxygen around the body. In addition, they are also required for proper nerve transmission and a shortfall of any of them will exacerbate any condition that affects the nervous system such as diabetic neuropathy.

B Vitamins

All the B vitamins work together. If a vitamin B supplements is being taken, then it is best to take a Balanced B Complex supplement. That way a person can be assured that they are getting their B vitamins in the correct ratios.

If more of a particular B vitamin is needed, then this can be taken in addition to the Balanced B Complex supplement. As always, make sure that whatever supplement is being taken it is from a natural source—not synthetic.

B vitamins are crucial for proper nerve function and a shortfall of any of them will exacerbate any nervous system condition, and especially diabetic neuropathy.

B1 (Thiamine)

Thiamine works with other B vitamins to break down food. It also keeps nerves and muscles in good order. The lack of this important vitamin in the body can lead to neuropathy, and on the other hand, thiamine (thiamin) can be an effective pain treatment for some types of diabetic neuropathy.

In addition, Thiamine is important for maintaining energy levels, for brain function and for good digestion. In addition it assists the body to utilize protein.

It is found in pork, vegetables, milk, cheese, peas, fresh and dried fruit, eggs, wholegrain breads and some breakfast cereals.

The Recommended Daily Allowance (RDA):
1.2mg (USA) 1.1mg (UK).

Vitamin B2 (Riboflavin)

Riboflavin helps maintain the skin, mucous membranes, eyes and the nervous system. It assists in producing steroids and red blood cells and helps the body to absorb iron from food.

It is found in many foods including milk, eggs, breakfast cereals, mushrooms and rice. Riboflavin can be destroyed by ultra violet light so these foods should be kept out of direct sunlight.

The Recommended Daily Allowance (RDA):
1.3mg (USA) 1.4mg (UK).

Vitamin B3 (Niacin)

Niacin like other B vitamins helps convert proteins, fats and carbohydrates into energy as well as keeping the digestive and nervous system healthy. It also helps in balancing blood sugar as well as lowering cholesterol levels. There are two types—nicotinic acid and nicotinamide. They're water soluble so they are needed every day.

Niacin is found in beef, pork, chicken, wheat flour, maize flour, milk and eggs.

The Recommended Daily Allowance (RDA):
16mg (USA) 16mg (UK).

Vitamin B5 (Pantothenic Acid)

Pantothenic acid also helps release the energy from food. It is also used by the adrenal glands to produce stress hormones during periods of physical and psychological stress.

Pantothenic Acid is found in most meat and vegetables especially chicken, beef, potatoes, porridge oats, tomatoes, kidney, eggs, broccoli, whole grains and rice. Some breakfast cereals are fortified with it.

The Recommended Daily Allowance (RDA):
5mg (USA) 6mg (UK).

Vitamin B6 (Pyridoxine)

Pyridoxine is necessary for metabolizing the amino acids in proteins, the formation of antibodies and red blood cells, and for maintaining a healthy digestive and nervous system.

Pyridoxine is found in pork, turkey, chicken, bread, cod and whole cereals such as wheat germ, oatmeal and rice. It is also contained in

milk, vegetables, eggs, soy milk, peanuts, potatoes and some breakfast cereals.

The Recommended Daily Allowance (RDA):
1.3mg (USA) 1.4mg (UK).

Vitamin B7 (Biotin)

Biotin is very important in childhood. It helps the body utilize essential fats and is also important for healthy hair, skin and nails. It
also helps turn food into energy as well as being involved in amino
acid metabolism. Since its water soluble, it is needed in the daily diet
because it can't be stored.

Biotin is found in a great many foods including kidney, egg yolk
and some fruits and vegetables, whole grains, and dried mixed fruit.

The Recommended Daily Allowance (RDA):
30mcg (USA) 50mcg (UK).

Vitamin B9 (Folic acid)

Known as folate in its natural form, it works with B12 to form
healthy blood cells and helps reduce the risk of defects in babies such
as spina bifida.

Folic Acid is found in small amounts in numerous foods but rich
sources are breakfast cereals, some types of bread and fruits such as
oranges and bananas. It is also found in broccoli, Brussels sprouts,
asparagus, peas, rice and chickpeas.

The Recommended Daily Allowance (RDA):
400mcg (USA) 200mcg (UK).

Vitamin B12 (Cyanocobalamin)

Vitamin B12 helps make red blood cells and generally keeps the
nervous system in optimum condition. It helps release energy from
the food that is eaten and it also helps process B9 (folic acid). It deals
with the effects of tobacco smoke as well as other toxins in the body.
A vitamin B12 deficiency can result in anemia. A long term deficiency of B12 can lead to damage of the nervous system. As a person
ages, it becomes more difficult to absorb B12.

It is found in fish, meat, poultry and dairy foods. Since it is not
found in vegetables, fruit or grains, vegans or vegetarians may find
they are deficient in it.

The Recommended Daily Allowance (RDA):
2.4mcg (USA) 2.5mcg (UK).

Because of the importance of B12 to a healthy nervous system, research done into combining B12, B6 and B9 vitamins has shown promising results in treating diabetic neuropathy.

A significant number of medications, which are prescribed to diabetics, have the effect of preventing significant absorption of vitamin B12, even when the recommended daily allowance (RDA) is consumed. Therefore, vitamin supplementation may become necessary.

Homocysteine

Homocysteine—a naturally occurring amino acid produced as part of the methylation process in the body, is found in high levels in some people with diabetic neuropathy. It is not usually found when there is an adequate supply of vitamin B6, B9 and B12 in the body.

Various factors are thought to raise levels of homocysteine; including poor diet, poor lifestyle, smoking and high coffee and alcohol consumption, various prescription drugs, diabetes, rheumatoid arthritis and a compromised thyroid function. Raised levels of homocysteine are also associated with potential health risks such as cardiovascular and Alzheimer's diseases, as well as various chronic inflammatory diseases and some intestinal disorders such as celiac and Crohn's diseases.

Vitamin C

Vitamin C is a water soluble, antioxidant vitamin which helps protect the body cells and keeps them healthy, as well as helping absorb iron from food. It is also used by the adrenal glands to produce hormones and helps to maintain healthy teeth and gums, cartilage, blood vessels and bones.

Vitamin C is found in low level in diabetic individuals. Researchers believe this is not due to individual sufferers not taking in enough vitamin C. In a diabetic condition, proper vitamin C consumption may occur, but the way that diabetes works in the body seems to have a negative impact on the many health benefits vitamin C offers.

Vitamin C is crucial for supporting the immune and nervous systems, both of these systems are compromised if an individual has diabetes. Extra care needs to be taken to ensure that an adequate intake of natural sources such as fruits and vegetables is consumed. If this is not possible, vitamin C supplementation will be necessary.

It is found in fruits such as oranges and kiwi fruit, as well as peppers, broccoli, Brussels sprouts and sweet potatoes.

Compared to other vitamins the body needs quite a lot of vitamin C every day—minimum 60 mg. However, higher doses are beneficial—up to 2000 mg. It may cause a loose bowel if taken excessively, but this will cease if the dose is reduced. Note! This is not a toxic condition.

The Recommended Daily Allowance (RDA):
90mg (USA) 80mg (UK).

Vitamin D
Vitamin D helps regulate the amounts of calcium and phosphorous in the body. These substances keep teeth and bones healthy. In addition, calcium is important in cases of proximal neuropathy.

It is only found in a small number of foods such as liver, oily fish and egg yolk. Other sources include margarine, cheese, butter, breakfast cereals and fortified milk. Most of the vitamin D in the human body is made in the skin because of its reaction to sunlight. Incidentally, most people—and especially children—lack vitamin D either through a lack of sun exposure, or it is lacking in the diet.

In children, vitamin D is important for proper growth and development. It is also important for the synthesis of calcium. If a female is pregnant or breast-feeding then they should supplement with vitamin D. Older people especially should take a vitamin D supplement. Individuals should also take it if they eat no meat or oily fish, rarely go outdoors or cover up when they do.

The Recommended Daily Allowance (RDA):
15mcg (USA) 5mcg (UK).

Vitamin E
Vitamin E is a fat soluble vitamin which is needed to help maintain a lot of the tissues in the body especially the eyes, skin and liver. As it is an antioxidant vitamin, it stops the lungs getting damaged by polluted air and it also helps in the production of red blood cells.

Diabetes can lead to a naturally low-level of vitamin E. Therefore, taking a daily supplement of this vitamin can prove to be beneficial. This is evidenced by research which has shown that vitamin E supplements consumed on a daily basis improves nerve transmission in individuals diagnosed with type 2 diabetes, in addition to reducing symptoms of peripheral neuropathy.

The richest sources of vitamin E are from plant oils such as soy, corn and olive oil as well as seeds, nuts, wheat germ, green leafy vegetables, egg yolk and olives.

The Recommended Daily Allowance (RDA):
15mg (USA) 12mg (UK).

Chapter 7
The Magic of Minerals

Every time a person moves their arms, blink their eyes, turn their head—they are using minerals. Minerals are not produced by the body, they are obtained from food that is eaten; therefore minerals are important for almost every body function. Calcium, magnesium and phosphorus are essential for bones and teeth. Nerve transmissions essential for brain and muscle actions depend on calcium, magnesium, sodium and potassium. Chromium is essential for controlling blood sugar levels—especially for people with diabetes. Zinc—an antioxidant mineral is essential as a free radical scavenger, also for body development as well as repair and renewal. Zinc and selenium—another antioxidant mineral supports the immune system.

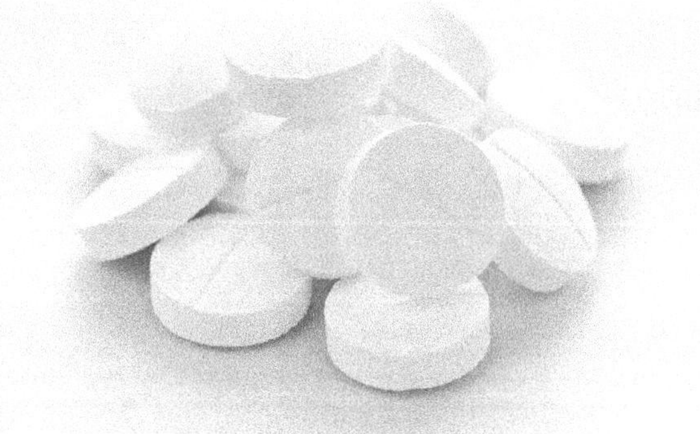

There are two types of minerals—macro or essential minerals, and trace minerals which are needed in very tiny amounts by the body.

As mentioned above, they have three main functions:

- Building strong bones and teeth
- Controlling body fluids inside and outside cells
- Converting food into energy

The main macro or essential minerals are:

- Calcium
- Iron
- Magnesium

- Phosphorus
- Potassium
- Sodium
- Sulfur

The trace elements are:

- Boron
- Cobalt
- Copper
- Chromium
- Germanium
- Iodine
- Manganese
- Molybdenum
- Selenium
- Silicon
- Zinc

Let us have a look in more detail at the important things that minerals and trace elements do in the body.

Boron

This trace element assists the body in making the best use of fats, glucose, estrogen and other minerals such as copper, calcium and magnesium. It occurs widely in plants, oceans, rocks and soil and can be found in green vegetables, fruit and nuts.

There is no Recommended Daily Allowance for Boron.

Calcium

Calcium is one of the most crucial minerals the body needs. As well as building strong teeth and bones, it is important in regulating muscle contractions which includes the heartbeat. It also ensures that blood clots normally when an individual receive a cut. It is also an important mineral for maintaining the correct acid / alkaline balance.

The main sources of calcium are milk, cheese and dairy products as well as green leafy vegetables such as cabbage broccoli, and okra (ladies' fingers). It is also found in soy beans, tofu, nuts, and bread made with fortified flour, as well as fish, such as sardines and pilchards when the bones are eaten.

When taking calcium as a supplement, it is preferable to take it in a combination form of calcium and magnesium. Vitamin D should also be in the formula as it helps with the absorption of calcium. Also important is phosphorus, which works with calcium, boron, copper, and zinc (an antioxidant mineral).

Calcium supplements on their own can cause constipation in some people. Magnesium helps to counteract the constipation effect of the calcium. As separate supplements, a person should take approximately half the amount of magnesium to what they are taking of calcium.

Middle-aged women as well as elderly men and women and those persons with a family history of osteoporosis, and white and Asian women between the ages of 11–35 can really benefit from an adequate calcium supplementation program.

Diabetics who suffer from proximal neuropathy should consider taking a calcium supplement. Proximal neuropathy causes a weakening of the muscles, and calcium is excellent at strengthening muscles as well as assisting in muscle contractions.

The Recommended Daily Allowance (RDA):
1000mg (USA) 800mg (UK).

Coral Calcium

Elsewhere in this book I have mentioned how the Western diet is acid forming which can lead to a condition called acidosis. Well, coral calcium is naturally alkaline, so it can be really important for those people who want to keep their pH levels within the normal range. Coral Calcium is especially important for females as it helps support mineral levels in the female body, especially in regard to natural hormone fluctuations.

As well as supplying important calcium to the body, any formulation should also contain magnesium as these two minerals help each other. Vitamin D should be in the formula too as it aids in the absorption of calcium.

There is no Recommended Daily Allowance for Coral Calcium.

Chromium

Chromium helps to regulate insulin in the body—which is especially important for individuals suffering from diabetes—and therefore has an effect on how much energy is obtained from the food that is eaten. It helps to reduce food cravings and improves lifespan. It is also important for proper heart function.

This trace element can be found in soil, air, water, animals and plants. In food it is found in meat, whole grains, spices and lentils.

The Recommended Daily Allowance (RDA):
35mcg (USA) 40mcg (UK).

Cobalt

Cobalt forms part of the structure of vitamin B12 which I discussed in the previous chapter. It is found widely in the environment. Fish, nuts, leafy green vegetables such as spinach, broccoli and cereals containing oats are all good food sources.

Basically, to get enough cobalt an individual needs to make sure they get enough vitamin B12.

There is no Recommended Daily Allowance for cobalt.

Copper

Copper is important in the production of both red and white blood cells. It also causes the release of iron to form hemoglobin, which is an iron-containing protein attached to red blood cells. This transports oxygen from the lungs to the rest of the body. Hemoglobin binds with oxygen in the lungs, which it then exchanges for carbon dioxide at the cellular level. It then transports the carbon dioxide back to the lungs to be exhaled.

Copper helps in child growth, the development of the brain and nervous system and producing strong bones. In addition, it assists in maintaining healthy skin and hair color and is also used to diminish the effects of inflammation associated with rheumatoid arthritis, and diabetic neuropathy.

It is found in nuts, shellfish and meat offal.

The Recommended Daily Allowance (RDA):
900mcg (USA) 1mg (UK).

Germanium

Many of the important herbs and medicinal plants traditionally used in healing, including ginseng, garlic, comfrey, and aloe vera, all contain substantial amounts of germanium. The therapeutic benefits of these herbs may be linked to the high amounts of germanium they contain.

Germanium also has antioxidant potential, and provides energy from carbohydrates in the diet. It is also found in a wide range of foods including beans, tomato juice, oysters and tuna, as well as those sources mentioned above.

Germanium comes in two forms—organic and inorganic. Inorganic germanium supplements have been withdrawn from sale because in this form they can damage the nervous system, liver and kidneys. The best organic supplements traditionally come from Japan where much of the research work has been done, particularly as a cancer preventative.

There is no Recommended Daily Allowance for germanium.

Iodine

Iodine helps make thyroid hormones which keep cells healthy and regulate the body's metabolic rate. It is found in seawater, seaweed, Black Walnut, rocks and soil as well as cow's milk. Fish and shellfish are especially rich in it. But it's also found in plant foods such as cereals and grains but this depends to a large extent on the amount of iodine found in the soils where those plants are grown.

Every cell in the body needs iodine. Interestingly, if a small amount of this brown liquid is put on the back of the hand it will have disappeared within 24 hours. In fact it will have been absorbed by the body's cells which "line up" to get a "fix" of this important mineral.

Inflammation is one of the greatest threats to the human body. And it is associated with diabetic neuropathy. It is often a precursor to more serious health conditions developing. Iodine is very effective in reducing inflammation in the body and thus helping to protect the body systems.

The Recommended Daily Allowance (RDA):
150mcg (USA) 150mcg (UK).

Iron

This is another of those essential minerals just about everyone has heard of. It is vital in the production of red blood cells to move oxygen around the body. The traditional way to get iron into the body systems was through organ meat such as liver. But there are plenty of other sources such as beans, nuts, dried fruit, whole grains, breakfast cereals, soybean flour and most green leafed vegetables, like water cress, curly kale and Brussels sprouts.

A lot of people think that spinach is a good source, but the problem is that spinach contains a substance which makes it harder for the body to absorb the iron from it. Strangely enough, both tea and coffee also contain substances which bind together with iron and make it more difficult for it to be absorbed. So cutting down on tea and coffee could boost iron levels in the body.

On the other hand, eating foods rich in vitamin C at the same time as foods containing iron from non-meat sources might actually help with iron absorption. So fruit juice with breakfast cereal or beans might prove beneficial.

Women who lose a lot of blood during their menstrual cycle may need iron supplements.

Women need more iron than men—around 14.8 mg as opposed to 8.7 mg for men.

The Recommended Daily Allowance (RDA):
8mg (USA) 14mg (UK).

Magnesium

Magnesium helps convert food to energy and makes sure that the parathyroid glands (which produce hormones to promote bone health) are working normally. It is also important for bones and teeth, as well as for the heart and nervous system. It is important for calcium uptake as well as being an anti-inflammatory mineral.

Magnesium can be obtained from nuts and green leafy vegetables as well as bread, meat, fish and dairy products.

The Recommended Daily Allowance (RDA):
400mg (USA) 375mg (UK).

Manganese

The trace element manganese helps activate over twenty enzymes in the body which assist in such things as food digestion. It is often found in supplements. It is also important for healthy bone formation, cartilage, tissues and nerve function, and is therefore an excellent mineral in case of diabetic neuropathy.

It occurs in bread, nuts, cereals and green vegetables such as peas and runner beans. Perhaps its main source for a lot of people is tea, drunk without milk.

The Recommended Daily Allowance (RDA):
2.3mg (USA) 2mg (UK).

Molybdenum

This is actually a heavy metal but as a trace element it's vital in activating those enzymes which produce and repair genetic material. It helps purge the body of waste protein by-products as well as detoxifying the body of free radicals, petroleum by-products and sulphites.

It is found in a lot of different foods, especially those vegetables which grow above ground such as peas, broccoli, spinach and cauliflower. It also occurs in nuts, tinned vegetables and oats.

The Recommended Daily Allowance (RDA):
45mcg (USA) 50mcg (UK).

Nickel

Nickel not only regulates the amount of iron in the body but it also plays a role in the production of red blood cells. It's important to note that one in ten people have an allergy to nickel so that if they come into contact with coins or jewelry containing it they may come out in a rash. The same can happen if an individual takes supplements containing nickel and have an allergy.

Nickel is very widespread in the environment and lentils, nuts and oats are good sources.

There is no Recommended Daily Allowance for nickel.

Phosphorous

Phosphorous has a number of important functions such as building strong bones and teeth and helping to release food energy. It is a component of DNA and RNA, as well as helping to maintain the acid/alkaline balance of the body.

It is found in dairy foods, fish, poultry, bread, rice and oats.

The Recommended Daily Allowance (RDA):
700mg (USA) 700mg (UK).

Potassium

Potassium controls the balance of fluids in the body and it may also help to reduce blood pressure. Potassium makes it possible for essential nutrients to move into body cells, and for waste products to be eliminated from them. It is also involved in insulin secretion to control blood sugar which supplies energy to the body. It is therefore important for diabetic sufferers.

Fruit such as bananas are rich in it as are vegetables, pulses, nuts, seeds, milk, fish, shellfish, beef, chicken, turkey and bread.

The Recommended Daily Allowance (RDA):
4700mg (USA) 2000mg (UK).

Selenium

Selenium plays a key role in the function of the immune system, in the production of thyroid hormones and in reproduction. It's also a key player in the body's antioxidant defense system which prevents damage to cells and tissue. It is an antioxidant mineral and works with vitamin E.

Brazil nuts, bread, fish, meat and eggs are all rich sources.

The Recommended Daily Allowance (RDA):
55mcg (USA) 55mcg (UK).

Silicon

More well-known for the chips in computers and other electrical gadgets, silicon helps maintain strong bones and helps keep connective tissue healthy.

It is found in grains such as barley, oats and rice as well as in fruit and vegetables.

There is no Recommended Daily Allowance (RDA) for silicon.

Sodium chloride

Better known as salt. There has been a lot of discussion in the media and in government concerning the tendency for people to eat too much of it, especially in such things as processed foods, which often have very high levels added. Indeed most people do eat too much. But it is a vital substance in keeping the fluids in the body well balanced. And because it is a central ingredient of the juices in the stomach and intestines it helps in the digestion of food.

Salt is found in low levels in virtually all foods. On average most people eat around 9.5 grams a day.

The Recommended Daily Allowance (RDA):
1500mg (USA) 800mg (UK).

Sulfur

Sulfur's functions include the production of tissue such as cartilage. It is involved in many key body functions such as reducing inflammation, pain from arthritis and diabetic neuropathy, as well as detoxification of the body.

Sulfur is also a constituent of keratin and collagen which are found in hair, skin and nails. Therefore sulfur compounds are beneficial for these three areas. One of the best forms of sulfur is the supplement MSM (methyl sulfonyl methane).

The therapeutic dose according to research into pain relief using MSM is a daily concentration between 1,500mg—3,000mg.

There is no Recommended Daily Allowance (RDA) for sulfur.

Tin

Very little research has been done on tin and its role in human health. One study showed psychological benefits of decreased depression and fatigue and an increase in positive mood and well-being in some study recipients, while others experienced a reduction in headaches, asthma, insomnia and general levels of pain.

Tin is available in small amounts from virtually all fruits and vegetables. It is absorbed by plants from the soil. How much is found in food depends on the levels in the soil where the plants are grown.

There is no Recommended Daily Allowance (RDA) for tin.

Vanadium

Some interesting animal studies indicate that vanadium may help to normalize glucose levels—which could potentially be good news for diabetic sufferers. The animal studies also indicate that vanadium could enhance athletic performance, and lower blood pressure. However, beneficial effects have yet to be conclusively proven in human studies.

Vanadium is a trace mineral that is essential for maintaining a healthy body. Vanadium is an opposite of molybdenum, which is another trace mineral, in that it works in tandem with it. Together, the two minerals help keep each other in balance and provide several health benefits to humans.

In animal and human studies it has been found that vanadium helped to reduce blood sugar levels and also increased insulin sensitivity in those individuals with type 1 and type 2 diabetes.

Food sources are seafood, cereals, mushrooms, parsley, corn, and soy.

There is no Recommended Daily Allowance (RDA) for vanadium.

Zinc

Zinc is an antioxidant mineral that helps make new cells and enzymes. It also functions with vitamins A and E to manufacture thyroid hormones.

It helps to process protein, fats and carbohydrates from foods and also with the healing of wounds.

Zinc is an important mineral in appetite control and a deficiency can cause a loss of taste and smell, thus creating a need for stronger tasting foods (which tend to be sweeter, saltier and more fattening.)

It is found in things like meat, shellfish, milk, dairy foods and cereals.

The Recommended Daily Allowance (RDA):
11mg (USA) 15mg (UK).

Zinc Lozenges

Zinc is often combined with Echinacea and Licorice Root (as a natural sweetener) to treat the effects of a sore throat or other mouth infections. It also supplies excellent immune system support.

Chapter 8

Essential Fatty Acids (EFA's)

Essential Fatty Acids are so called because they have to be obtained from the diet—the body cannot make them itself. There are two essential fatty acids: omega-3 and omega-6. These two are the building blocks that make the twenty fatty acids that the body needs for good health. I discuss these two oils, along with several others in greater detail, later in this chapter.

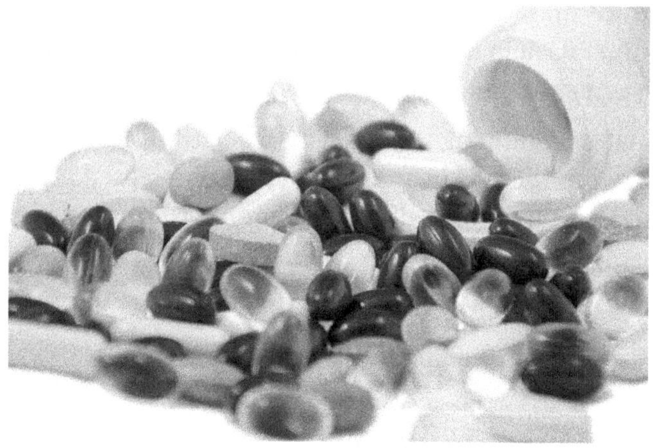

Essential fatty acids are important for the manufacture of cell membranes as well as important hormones and neurotransmitters—chemical substances that pass messages between different cells which tell the body what to do.

They are also involved in the manufacture of prostaglandins in the body. These hormone-like substances help control many different activities. Some of these activities include such things as inflammation, pain control, and unbelievably, some cause swelling and some reduce swelling. They are involved in allergic reactions, blood clotting and the manufacture of other hormones.

Prostaglandins also have a role to play in controlling blood pressure, heart and kidney function, body temperature in addition to being involved in the digestive system.

Being natural blood thinners, fatty acids help prevent blood clots, which can trigger a heart attack or stroke.

Arthritis, instances of diabetic neuropathy and autoimmune diseases can be relieved by the natural anti-inflammatory compounds found in essential fatty acids.

An individual who experiences skin problems or has dull or brittle hair, or nails that split easily, or has dandruff or eczema, may have a diet that could be lacking in essential fatty acids.

Essential Fatty Acids have an important role to play in good digestive and intestinal systems health. They help maintain cell stability in addition to increasing the thickness of cells lining the intestinal tract, as well as the villi which enhances the absorption of nutrients. All this leads to better digestion and improved health.

DHA—an omega-3 fatty acid is the most plentiful fat in the brain. It is important for ensuring that chemical messages pass effectively between the brain cells. Copious quantities of omega-3 fatty acids are also found in the retina of the eye.

Omega-3 fatty acids are also found in high concentrations in breast milk. Babies require it for their brain growth and vision development.

Low levels of essential fatty acids in the diet have been linked to vision problems, mood swings, diabetes, memory loss and dementia.

So how much essential fatty acid should an individual take? It all depends on such factors as: what type of diet a person has? The typical Western diet is very rich in omega-6 essential fatty acids which can cause a hormone imbalance leading to various health problems.

The ideal ratio is one portion of omega-3 to 5 portions of omega-6. In the typical Western diet which is high in saturated fat the ratio is often one portion of omega-3 to 20 portions of omega-6. To counteract this imbalance it might be a good idea to use the following formula. For every portion of omega 6, take 2 portions of omega-3. If an individual finds it difficult to achieve this with their diet, then they can consider taking an omega-3 supplement. Incidentally, there is no Recommended Daily Allowance (RDA) for essential fatty acids. Men may need to take more than women. Also, if a person suffers from stress, diabetic neuropathy or other health problems then more may be needed.

Essential Fatty Acid Supplements

Black Currant Oil

Black currant oil is a rich source of omega-3 (linolenic essential fatty acid (EFA), alpha linolenic acid (ALA), and omega-6 gamma linoleic essential fatty acid (GLA), along with other important poly-unsaturated fatty acids.

Fatty acids are involved in most body functions, from maintaining body temperature to providing a cushion for and protecting body tissue as well as protecting the nervous system and creating energy.

Interestingly, before the discovery of the benefits of black currant oil, the only other known sources of GLA were mother's milk and evening primrose oil.

CLA

CLA, or conjugated linoleic acid, is a mixture of essential fatty acids that are important for maintaining healthy body functions.

CLA helps to sustain lean muscle mass as well as enhancing the burning of fat, which makes it a useful product in a weight-loss regime, in addition to instances of proximal neuropathy.

DHA

DHA (docosahexaenoic acid) is an omega-3 fatty acid sourced from oily fish such as herring, mackerel, salmon, and sardines that is absorbed into the fatty perimeter of cells where it exerts its biochemical properties. DHA offers many benefits. It supports and protects the nervous system and supports brain and eye health as well as the health of the skin.

Evening Primrose Oil

Evening Primrose is a plant that grows throughout the US and Europe. The plant grows close to the ground and the oil is found in the plants seeds. This oil is rich in gamma linolenic acid (GLA, an omega-6 essential fatty acid).

The oil is traditionally used to treat various skin conditions such as eczema and dermatitis and to alleviate breast tenderness from pre-menstrual syndrome (PMS).

Evening Primrose Oil seems to be more effective for the above conditions when taken with an omega-3 supplement from fish oil (derived from oily cold water fish such as salmon, tuna, mackerel and sardines) to create a healthy body balance.

Evening Primrose Oil is also used in the manufacture of some cosmetics and soap.

It is available as an oil or in capsule form. It should be kept out of direct sunlight and preferably stored in a refrigerator to prevent rancidity.

Flax Seed Oil

The Flax plant is a blue, flowering plant that is grown in Ireland and the western Canadian prairies. No part of the plant is wasted. The inner stems contain fibers that are made into linen for use in the manufacture of bedding as well as clothes. The oil-rich seeds of the plant, known as flax seed oil or linseed oil, are used for cattle feed, in the paint industry, and as a rich source of omega-3 and -6 essential fatty acids for human consumption. These natural essential fatty acids are used for the general well-being and support of most body systems.

Flax Seed is considered to be one of nature's richest sources of alpha-linolenic acid (ALA)—(an omega-3 fatty acid)—as well as containing omega-6 essential fatty acids. In addition, flax seed oil contains B vitamins, potassium, lecithin, magnesium, fiber, protein, and zinc.

It also contains Lignans which are a type of fiber that is changed by "friendly bacteria" in the gut into compounds that fight against cancer.

Krill Oil

Krill are tiny crustaceans that serve as a good food source for whales, seals, and other ocean mammals. They also provide a rich source of essential omega-3 fatty acids, including EPA and DHA.

Omega-3 essential fatty acids are important for cardiovascular and brain health as well as providing support for joints and the skin. Krill is a natural source of powerful antioxidant carotenoids.

Krill oil naturally contains phospholipids, which attach to omega-3 fatty acids, enhancing their absorption in the body. Phospholipids strengthen cell membranes as well as making them more elastic, which helps to keep toxins out and let nutrients and oxygen in.

Omega-3 Essential Fatty Acids

There are several different types of omega-3 essential fatty acids:

Alpha Linolenic Acid (ALA) good sources are: canola, flaxseed, rapeseed, soybeans, and walnuts.

Eicosapentaenoic acid (EPA) which is obtained from cold water, oily fish: herrings, salmon, sardines and tuna are good sources.

Docosahexaenoic acid (DHA) which is also obtained from cold water, oily fish: herrings, salmon, sardines and tuna are good sources.

Omega-3 is one of basic fats that the body obtains from foods. While many fats are harmful, omega-3 benefits the body and is especially important for the heart.

Omega-3 fatty acids contain natural anti-inflammatory compounds that can provide relieve to those people who suffer from rheumatoid arthritis, diabetic neuropathy, psoriasis, allergies, and other inflammatory diseases. It can also help reduce irritation and swelling.

The body uses omega-3 fatty acids as one of the primary building blocks of cell membranes, as well as being beneficial to the structural system and for lubricating the skin. In other words, it helps the skin stay supple and soft.

Omega-6 Essential Fatty Acids

There are several different types of omega-6 essential fatty acids:

Linoleic Acid (LA) good sources are corn oil, cottonseed oil, peanut oil, rice bran oil, safflower oil, Soybean oil and sunflower oil.

Arachidonic acid (AA) obtained from: dairy products, eggs, meat and peanut oil.

Gamma Linolenic Acid (GLA)—an oil blend, which provides omega-6 essential fatty acids (linoleic and gamma-linolenic acids). This is obtained mainly from plant based oils, such as: black currant oil, borage oil, and evening primrose oil. In addition, most of these oils also contain some linoleic acid (LA).

In the body, this oil blend can be converted into hormone-like substances that regulate many important body functions and processes. These substances may benefit circulatory system health and skin and joint health as well as enhance the immune and nervous systems.

GLA provides nutritional support to the female reproductive system, especially before menstruation when mild mood changes, breast tenderness, cramps, and swelling can occur.

Alpha Lipoic Acid

Alpha lipoic acid is a very powerful antioxidant fatty acid which is found in every cell of the body. The body utilizes it to convert glucose (blood sugar) into energy for normal body functions, and is therefore important for diabetic sufferers.

Alpha lipoic acid is able to function in both water and fat, unlike the more common antioxidants vitamins C which functions in water and vitamin E which functions in fat.

A unique feature of Alpha Lipoic Acid is that it can recycle antioxidants such as vitamin C and glutathione after they have been expended. Meaning, they can be used again to fulfil body functions. Glutathione is an important antioxidant that assists the body in eliminating harmful substances. Alpha lipoic acid enhances the formation of glutathione.

Although the body manufactures Alpha Lipoic Acid, it is also found in brewer's yeast, broccoli, Brussels sprouts, organ meats, peas, rice bran and spinach.

Alpha Lipoic Acid is also intimately involved in brain function by crossing the blood brain barrier (a wall of structural cells and tiny blood vessels) to protect nerve and brain tissue from the effects of free radical damage.

Other uses for Alpha Lipoic Acid include: supporting the body after chemotherapy, dietary deficiencies, alcoholism, diabetes, kidney disease, Lyme disease, shingles and thyroid disorders.

Alpha Lipoic Acid is available as a supplement in capsule form, and in studies the daily amount that was best tolerated by the body, and to supply adequate amounts was 600mg, taken on an empty stomach.

Lecithin

Lecithin is found in many food sources including cabbage, cauliflower, eggs, garbanzo beans, organic meat, seeds, soy beans, split peas and nuts. It is also manufactured by the body provided the correct nutrients are available for it to do so. Unfortunately this is not always the case with the average Western diet; therefore supplementation is almost always necessary. Supplements can be in either liquid or capsule form. Lecithin is non-toxic.

Lecithin is an important phospholipid which is needed and utilized by all body cells as well as the heart, liver and kidneys. As it is a fat itself, it adheres to cell and nerve linings, forming a slippery barrier to prevent cholesterol and other fats from sticking. This ensures that blood flows more freely. It is also important for supporting brain function, and for supporting the nervous system, especially in cases of diabetic neuropathy.

When Lecithin breaks down body fats, it then transports these fats to the liver and helps convert them into usable energy.

Chapter 9

Functions of the Nervous System

The nervous system is one of the key systems that can be adversely affected when a person suffers from diabetic neuropathy. Conditions such as pain, inflammation, stress, and depression are all linked to this debilitating disease. In this section, I have given an overview of the nervous system, and the important role it plays in good body health.

Basic Function

The basic function of the nervous system is to trigger and monitor all communication process in the body.

While the brain is the master controller, the nervous system also has local control points. For example, a burn reflex travels to and from the spinal cord, so a person would withdraw their hand before their brain knew what had happened.

There are three types of neurons: sensory neurons, which receive stimuli and carry impulses to the central nervous system (CNS); inter-neurons, which connect two or more neurons; and motor-neurons, which carry impulses away from the CNS to muscles or glands.

Impulses travel from one nerve cell to another across a synapse with the help of chemical transmitters. Among these are acetylcholine, nor-epinephrine and serotonin.

Neuron

A nerve cell that includes receiving and transmitting arms that link it to billions of nerve cells throughout the body.

Neurotransmitter

One of several types of chemical messengers.

Brain

As master controller (and weighing an average of three pounds), it uses 20 percent of the body's total energy supply to power an estimated 10 billion brain cells.

Central Nervous System

The brain and spinal cord

Peripheral Nervous System

A network of nerves branching out from the spinal cord throughout the body.

Common Problems Associated With The Nervous System:

- Headaches

- Insomnia

- Nervous disorders

- Depression

- Memory trouble

Lifestyle Suggestions:

- Eat regular, wholesome meals.

- Avoid smoking, alcohol and stimulants.

- Exercise regularly.

- Manage stress.

- Eat lots of green, leafy vegetables, fruits, whole grains and nuts.

Interesting Facts:

- Some nerve fibers can conduct nerve impulses as fast as 200 yards per second.

- Scientists are investigating evidence that dead nerve cells can be replaced by the body, a process once thought to be impossible.

- Prescriptions for antidepressants have increased over 100 percent in the last five years.

- To combat anxiety, a daily walk may be as effective as tranquilizers.

Supplements for Nervous System Health

Stress:
B Complex and Vitamin C

When the body is under stress, a B Complex vitamin supplement may be required along with vitamin C. B vitamins and vitamin C are water soluble and are easily depleted from the body, especially during stressful times. All the B vitamins work together so it is usually preferable to take a B Complex supplement and then top-up with individual B vitamins if required. The B vitamins and vitamin C are often referred to as the stress vitamins.

Depression:
St. John's Wort

This popular herb has gained national attention for its ability to alleviate mild to moderate depression. It contains an active constituent, hypericin, which appears to prolong the activity of serotonin (a neurotransmitter) in the brain. St. John's Wort may also lengthen the performance of dopamine and nor-epinephrine, two brain chemicals that are linked to depression. In Europe, many doctors prescribe this herb instead of prescription antidepressant drugs.

Note! You can find further details on Stress and Depression by reading my book *"An Easy Way to Understand Stress and Depression"*, which is available from the Kindle Store, or in print form from Amazon.com.

Mind Memory Loss, Poor Memory:
Ginkgo Biloba

Ginkgo Biloba promotes increased circulation. It also dilates blood vessels and bronchioles to improve circulation and oxygenation of cells. It also has scientifically proven nervous-system benefits in addition to improving memory function.

In Summary

It is unfortunate, that even if the underlying diabetic condition has been successfully reversed or controlled, some of the effects which have been caused are unrepairable. Instances of diabetes in an advanced state can cause very serious damage to the nervous system, which then has the effect of damaging surrounding muscle and organ tissue.

It is important to remember that the symptoms and consequently the effects of this neuropathy can be managed or minimized. There are natural and pharmaceutical options available to assist in reducing the incidence and intensity of any symptoms experienced.

Important research is ongoing to discover various methods of overcoming present damage.

In the meantime, the best cure for diabetic neuropathy symptoms is similar to that which caused the diabetic condition, and that is to make better more healthy choices in relation to the diet and exercise.

About The Author

Brian B Jacques started in business at a young age, and over the ensuing years, he has developed several very successful businesses. But his main interest for the past 40 years has been in natural health research and publishing.

Brian has presented seminars worldwide on such diverse subjects as Health Related issues, Motivation and Personal Development. In addition he has written numerous books, newsletters and articles on these subjects.

His very popular series of Mini Health Books has circulated widely around the world, and many more titles are in preparation.

Brian is a highly motivated individual, so much so that in 1985 he received a UK Industrial Society award for his work in the Motivation and Personal Development fields.

Brian has the following mottos:

- If something does not work out for you, then don't give up, but keep trying, trying, trying until finally you succeed.
- Success or failure in any endeavor is in your own hands.

Brian and his wife divide their time between East Yorkshire, UK and Florida, USA.

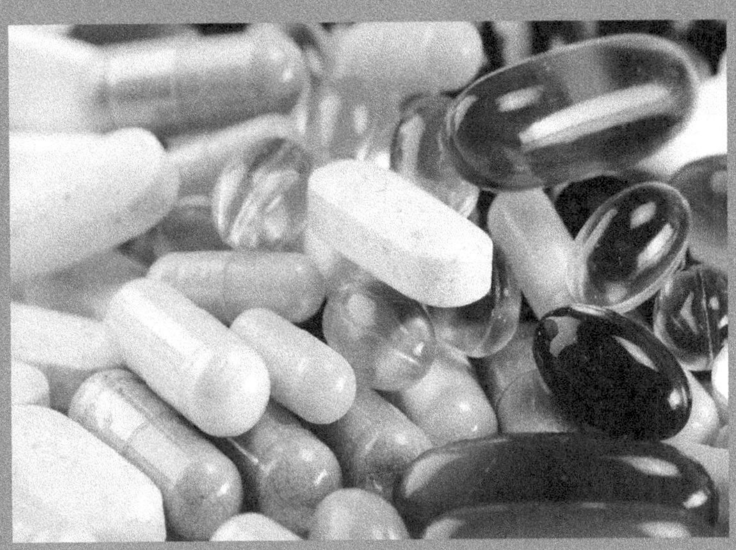